ANTI INFLAMMATORY DIET

Strengthening the Immune System with Natural Nutrition and Living in a State of Well-Being

SUSAN MULLER

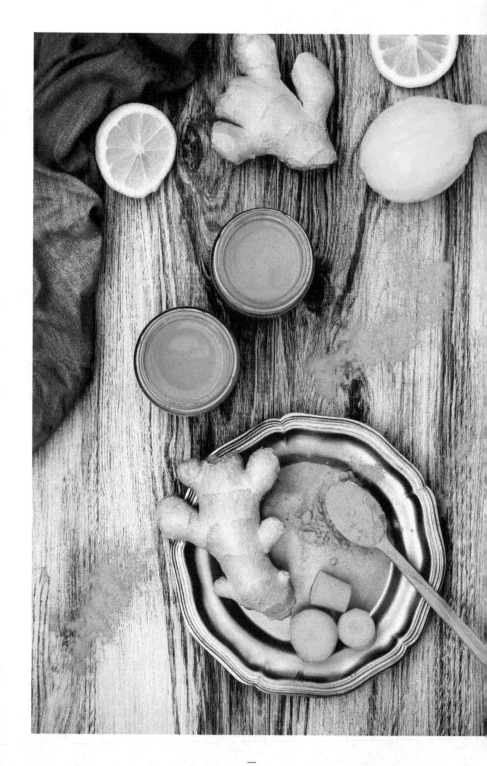

Table of Contents

Sommario

Introduction

The anti-inflammatory diet is a dietary regimen capable of counteracting chronic systemic inflammation, the main cause of the onset of chronic diseases of our century

The anti-inflammatory diet allows curing that state of general malaise that pervades and from which there seems to be no escape and can prevent the onset of diseases related to physiological aging. In addition, with an anti-inflammatory diet, you can keep under control the symptoms of the chronic disease that afflicts you, making the body more receptive to treatment.

An anti-inflammatory diet balanced on personal characteristics can

- reduce mitochondrial oxidative stress
- stimulate the liver to regenerate and cleanse itself of metabolic wastes
- modulate the release of inflammation mediators (e.g. prostaglandins, cytokines)
- inhibit the action of free radicals
- modulate the hormonal response
- promote weight loss where necessary

Weight loss is extremely important to amplify the anti-inflammatory process of the diet. The adipose tissue is an endocrine organ that releases bio-active molecules known as adipokines largely with pro-inflammatory activity.

An anti-inflammatory diet is built by focusing on reducing the intake of pro-inflammatory foods and increasing anti-inflammatory foods.

Among the anti-inflammatory foods it is important to favor:

- FRUITS AND VEGETABLES
- WHOLE GRAINS
- LEGUMES
- OMEGA 3: (DRIED FRUIT and SEEDS, ALGAE, FISH, EXTRA-VIRGIN OLIVE OIL)
- GREEN TEA
- DARK CHOCOLATE
- SPICES AND AROMATIC HERBS

Among the pro-inflammatory foods to limit and avoid:

- SUGAR
- REFINED CEREALS.
- INDUSTRIAL FOODS
- SUNFLOWERS and VEGETABLES
- MILK AND DAIRY PRODUCTS
- RED MEAT AND PROCESSED MEAT

It is also good to pay attention to cooking, preferring the simplest and "sweetest" (e.g. steam, oven), which do not impoverish the food but preserve its qualities. Therefore no high temperatures, barbecuing or grilling, or direct contact with fire.

Where necessary, to enhance the anti-inflammatory effect of the diet you can consider the use of quality supplements such as probiotics to restore the balance of the microbiome and correct intestinal dysbiosis or based on omega 3 or antioxidants (vitamin C, E, curcumin, selenium, carotenoids, coenzyme Q10, etc.).

Choose an anti-inflammatory diet is possible at all ages, associating it with an active lifestyle that includes

healthy aerobic physical activity (e.g. brisk walking, running, cycling, etc.) attention in the assumption of drugs, especially to the "self-medication practice relaxation techniques to combat stress (eg meditation).

The anti-inflammatory diet aims to "cure" a systemic inflammation of low degree but also to prevent it. It is a dietary regimen to be established from childhood and advisable for all those who are interested in the well-being of their body and want to prevent the onset of disease.

"Let food be your medicine and medicine be your food."

BREAKFAST

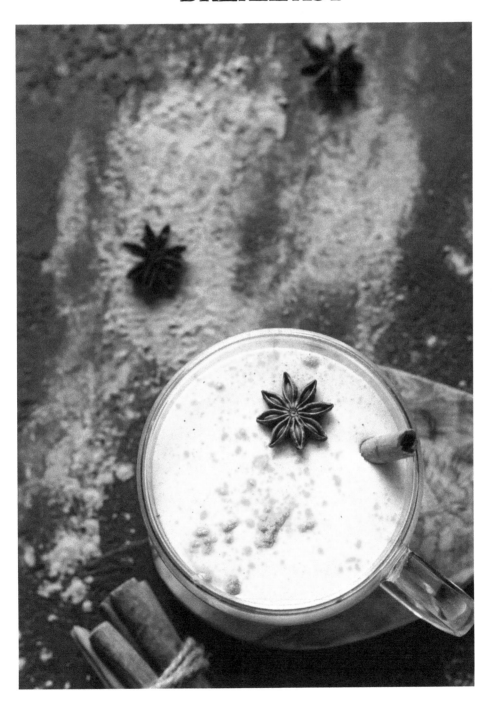

Apple Breakfast Dream

Ingredients:

2 cup raw walnuts

1 cup raw macadamia nuts

2 apples, peeled and diced

1 Tbsp coconut oil

1 Tbsp ground cinnamon

2 cup almond milk

1 14 oz can full fat coconut milk

Instructions:

Combine nuts and dates in a food processor until ground into a fine meal, about 1 minute; set aside.

Saute apples over medium heat in coconut oil until lightly browned, about 5 minutes.

Add nut mixture and cinnamon to apples and stir to incorporate, about 1 minute.

Reduce heat to low and add coconut and almond milk.

Stirring occasionally, let mixture cook uncovered until thickened, about 25 minutes.

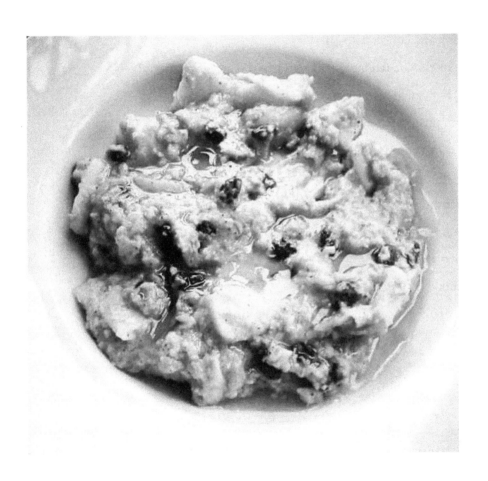

Divine Protein Muesli

Ingredients:

1 cup unsweetened unsulfured coconut flakes

1 tbsp chopped walnuts

1 tbsp raw almonds (~10)

1 tbsp chocolate chips (soy, dairy, and gluten free brand)

1/2 tsp cinnamon (Ceylon)

1 cup unsweetened almond milk

1 scoop hemp protein

Instructions:

In a medium bowl layer coconut flakes, walnuts, almonds, raisins and chocolate chips.

Sprinkle with cinnamon.

Pour cold almond milk over the muesli and eat with a spoon.

Paleo Garlic Breadsticks (Just Don't Eat Them All Yourself)

Ingredients:

1 1/3 cups almond flour

1/2 tsp salt

2 tbsp coconut oil, melted

3 tbsp coconut flour

1 clove garlic, minced

3 eggs, divided

1 tsp dried basil

1/2 tsp onion powder

1/2 tsp oregano

1/2 tsp baking powder

Ghee, for brushing

Instructions:

Whisk two eggs together in a small bowl and set aside. In a separate bowl, add the almond flour, baking powder, salt, and coconut oil and stir. Add the beaten eggs and stir to combine.

Add the coconut flour into the bowl, one tablespoon at a time. After each tablespoon let the dough rest for a minute as the flour absorbs. Add the next tablespoon and repeat until you have dough that can be easily kneaded.

Preheat the oven to 350 degrees F. Line a baking sheet with parchment paper. Roll out the dough onto a separate piece of parchment paper. Working in small handfuls, roll the dough into a long rope. Twist the dough into your shape of choice and place on the baking sheet. Bake for 10 minutes.

Whisk the remaining egg and add a dash of water. Remove the breadsticks from the oven and brush with the egg wash, and then the minced garlic, basil, onion powder and oregano. Return to the oven and bake for 4-5 minutes more, until golden. Brush with melted ghee before serving.

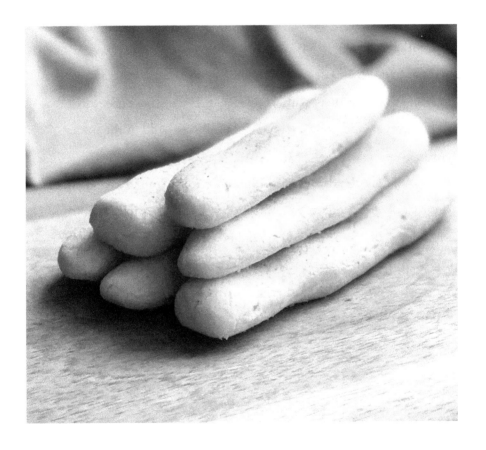

Homemade Strawberry Fruit Leather

Ingredients:

4 cups strawberries, hulled and chopped

2 tbsp honey

Instructions:

Preheat the oven to 170 degrees F or the lowest oven temperature setting. Line a baking sheet with a Silpat mat. Place strawberries in a medium saucepan and cook on low heat until soft. Add in the honey and stir to combine.

Use an immersion blender to puree the strawberries in the saucepan, or transfer to a blender and puree until smooth. Pour the mixture onto the Silpat-lined baking sheet and spread evenly with a spatula. Bake for 6-7 hours, until it peels away from the parchment.

Once cooled, peel the fruit leather off the mat and use a scissors to cut the fruit leather into strips. Roll up to serve, and store in an airtight container.

Coco Chocco Granola Recipe

Ingredients:

1 & 1/2 cup almonds

1 & 1/2 cup other nuts/seeds (or more almonds. I did a combo of pepitas, sunflower seeds and walnuts)

1 cup flax seed meal

1 cup flaked coconut (unsweetened)

Stevia to taste

1/2 tsp salt

1/3 cup Kelapo coconut oil, melted

1 egg

1/2 cup cacao nibs

Instructions:

Preheat oven to 300F and line a large rimmed baking sheet with parchment paper.

In the bowl of a food processor, combine almonds and other nuts or seeds. Pulse until mixture resembles coarse crumbs with some bigger pieces in there too. Transfer to a large bowl and add flax seed meal, flaked coconut, sweetener of choice, and salt.

Drizzle with coconut oil and stir to combine. Add egg, and toss until mixture begins to clump together. Stir in cacao nibs. Spread mixture evenly on prepared baking sheet and bake 20 minutes, stirring frequently. Remove and let cool.

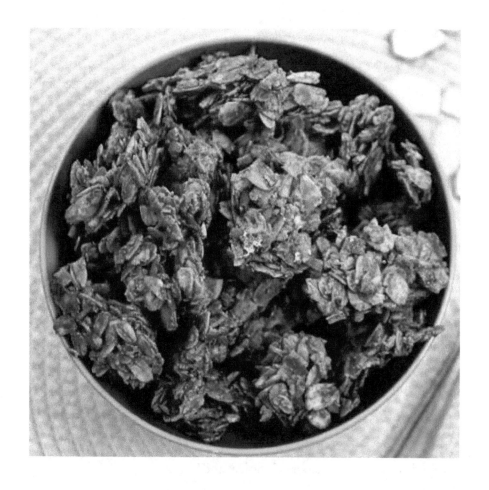

Cherry Almond Muesli Recipe

Ingredients:

3 cups slivered almonds

1 cup sunflower seeds

1 cup unsweetened shredded coconut

¼ teaspoon salt

2 tablespoons coconut oil, melted

Stevia

1 teaspoon vanilla extract

1 cup dried cherries

Instructions:

Preheat oven to 300 degrees.

Combine nuts, seeds, coconut and salt in large bowl. Combine coconut oil, honey and vanilla in a small bowl, and then stir into nut mixture until well combined.

Bake on a rimmed cookie sheet lined with parchment paper for 18 - 20 minutes, until just lightly browned.

Add the dried cherries and toss to combine. Cool completely before serving.

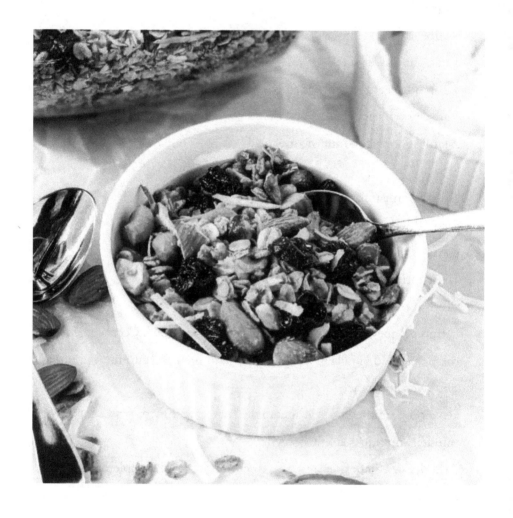

Homemade Strawberry Fruit Leather

Ingredients:

4 cups strawberries, hulled and chopped

2 tbsp honey

Instructions:

Preheat the oven to 170 degrees F or the lowest oven temperature setting. Line a baking sheet with a Silpat mat. Place strawberries in a medium saucepan and cook on low heat until soft. Add in the honey and stir to combine.

Use an immersion blender to puree the strawberries in the saucepan, or transfer to a blender and puree until smooth. Pour the mixture onto the Silpat-lined baking sheet and spread evenly with a spatula. Bake for 6-7 hours, until it peels away from the parchment.

Once cooled, peel the fruit leather off the mat and use a scissors to cut the fruit leather into strips. Roll up to serve, and store in an airtight container.

Healthier Chicken Nuggets Recipe

Ingredients:

1 chicken breast cut into bite size pieces

1 egg

1/4 cup almond flour breadcrumbs

seasoning

Instructions:

Mix the seasoning with the breadcrumbs (choose your seasoning, I have made them with Italian seasoning, spices, whatever my mood leads me to throw in), dip chicken pieces in egg then roll in the breadcrumbs and place on the mesh rack in the lower tier of the big boss (I am sure these would cook just fine in a regular oven).

This was enough chicken nuggets for two of us. I baked them in the big boss at 375F turning as they browned. It took about 18 minutes plus a few mins of prep. No oil was used and they surprisingly did not stick to the mesh tray (the ones with regular bread crumbs did stick).

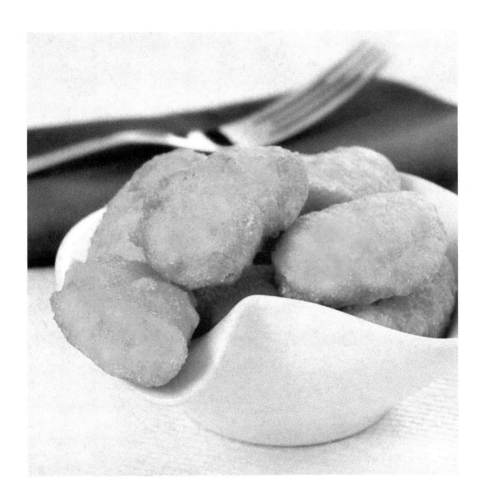

LUNCH

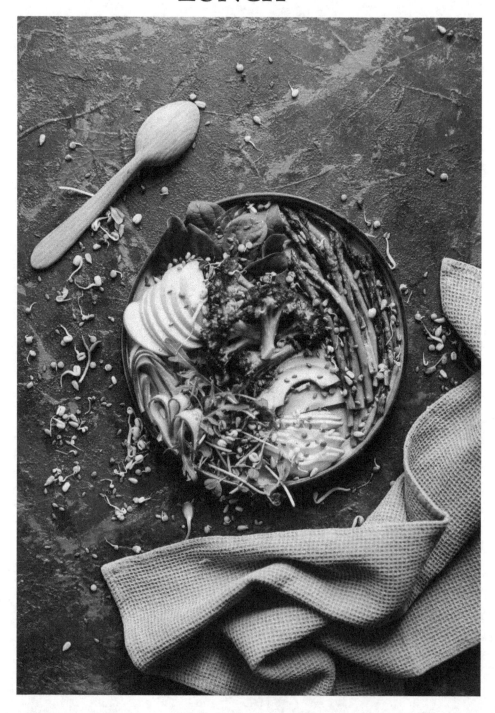

Avocado Tuna Salad

Ingredients:

2 tins high quality albacore tuna

1 avocado

1/4 of an onion chopped

juice of 1/2 a lime

2 Tbsp cilantro (or sub basil if you prefer)

some low sodium salt and pepper, to taste

Instructions:

Shred the tuna.

Add all of the other ingredients and mix.

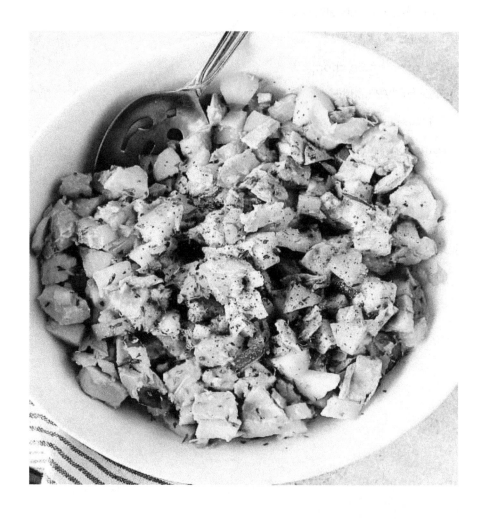

Macadamia Nut Chicken/Turkey Salad

Ingredients:

1lb chicken/turkey breast

1tsp macadamia nut oil, or oil of choice

few pinches of low sodium salt and pepper

1/2 cup macadamia nuts, chopped

1/2 cup diced celery

3 tbsp divine dressing

2 tbsp julienned basil

1 tbsp lemon juice

Instructions:

Preheat oven to 350. Place chicken breasts on sheet tray, drizzle will oil and a pinch of low sodium salt and pepper.

Bake for about 35 minutes until cooked through. Remove from oven and let cool.

In a large bowl shred chicken. Add nuts, celery, basil, mayo, lemon juice, and a pinch of low sodium salt and pepper. Gently stir until combined. Eat!

Divine Dressing:

Mix together, 4 Tbsp. chili powder, 1 tsp each garlic powder, onion powder, and oregano, 2 tsp each paprika and cumin, 4 tsp low sodium salt, and 1/8-1/4 tsp red pepper flakes. Add 1 cup olive oil and half cup rice vinegar.

Paleo Mini Meatloaves

Ingredients:

2 pounds ground meat – mixture of grass fed beef and/or pork and/or veal

10 ounces frozen, chopped spinach

1-2 teaspoons oil

1 medium onion, finely diced

6 ounces mushrooms, finely diced

2 carrots, grated or finely diced

4 eggs, lightly beaten

1/3 cup coconut flour

2 teaspoons salt

2 teaspoons pepper

2 teaspoons onion powder

1 teaspoon garlic powder

1 teaspoon dried thyme

1/4 teaspoon grated nutmeg

Instructions:

Preheat oven to 375 degrees F

Thaw the spinach, squeeze out the excess water and set aside.

Heat a pan on medium heat, add the oil and fry the onions and mushrooms until the onions are translucent and some of the liquid has cooked out of the mushrooms. Set aside to cool.

Place the ground meat in a large bowl, add the spinach, carrots, mushroom/onion mixture, beaten eggs, coconut flour and all the spices. Use your hands to combine it well but do not overmix. Fill 18 regular size muffin tins to the top with the meatloaf mixture. (Greasing the tins may be a good idea if the meat you're using is fairly lean) Cook for 20-25 minutes or until internal temperature reaches 160 degrees.

Allow to cool and use a knife to loosen meatloaves from sides of the pan before removing.

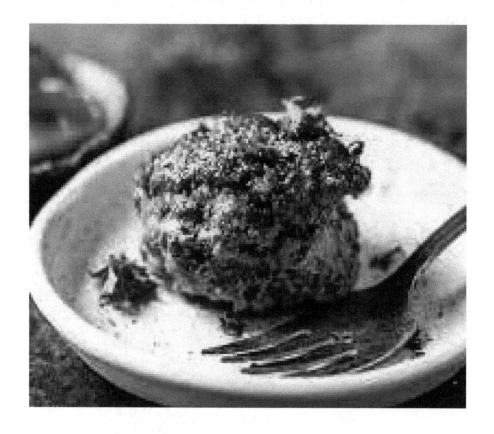

Eggplant Bolognese with Zucchini Noodles
(Low Carb)

Ingredients:

1 1/2 lbs. eggplant, diced

1/2 lb. ground beef

2 tbsp extra virgin olive oil

Salt and freshly ground pepper

1 large yellow onion, chopped

3 cloves garlic, minced

2 bay leaves

4 sprigs thyme

1 tbsp tomato paste

1/2 cup red wine

1 28-oz. can whole peeled plum tomatoes

6 leaves fresh basil, chiffonade

Instructions:

Heat the olive oil in a large pan over medium-high heat. Add in the onion and beef and sprinkle with salt and pepper. Cook for 8-10 minutes until the meat is browned. Stir in the eggplant, garlic, bay leaves, and thyme and sauté for an additional 15 minutes.

Once the eggplant is tender, stir in the tomato paste. Add the wine and scrape any browned bits off the bottom of the pan. Stir in the tomatoes and slightly crush with a spoon. Bring the mixture to a boil, then reduce the heat and simmer for 10 minutes, stirring occasionally. Adjust salt to taste. Serve warm garnished with fresh basil.

Kale and Red Pepper Frittata

Ingredients:

1 tbsp coconut oil

1/2 cup chopped red pepper

1/3 cup chopped onion

3 slices crispy bacon, chopped

2 cups chopped kale, de-stemmed and rinsed

8 large eggs

1/2 cup almond or coconut milk

Salt and pepper to taste

Instructions:

Preheat oven to 350 degrees. In a medium bowl, whisk the eggs and milk together. Add salt and pepper. Set aside.

In a non-stick skillet, heat about a tablespoon of coconut oil over medium heat. Add onion and red pepper and sauté for 3 minutes, until onion is translucent. Add kale and cook until it wilts, about 5 minutes. Add eggs to the pan mixture, along with the bacon. Cook for about 4 minutes until the bottom and edges of the frittata start to set.

Put frittata in the oven and cook for 10-15 minutes until the frittata is cooked all the way through. Slice and serve.

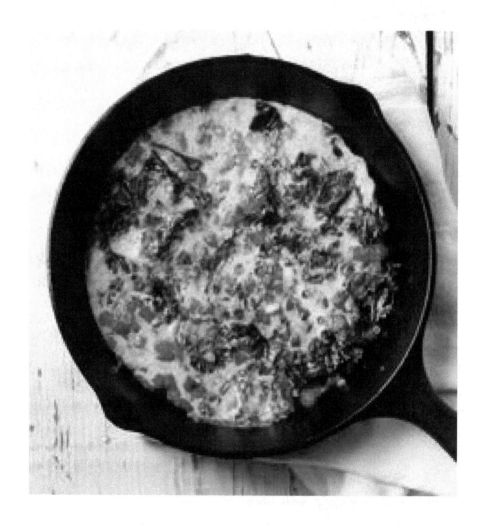

The Best Homemade Ranch Dressing Ever

Ingredients:

1/2 cup Paleo mayo (see below)

1/2 cup coconut milk

1/2 tsp onion powder

1 tsp garlic powder

1 tsp dill

Salt and freshly ground pepper, to taste

Instructions:

Whisk all ingredients together to combine. Season with salt and pepper to taste. Store in an airtight container in the refrigerator for up to a week.

Mayo recipe

1 egg, room temperature

2 tbsp lemon juice or apple cider vinegar

1/2 tsp salt

1/2 tsp dry mustard

1 cup light olive oil*

In a tall glass (if using an immersion blender) or a blender, place the egg and lemon juice. Let come to room temperature, about one hour. Add the salt and mustard. Blend ingredients. While blending, very slowly pour in the olive oil. Blend until it reaches desired consistency. Store in the refrigerator for up to a week.

*It's important to use a light olive oil, not full flavour, for mayonnaise. You could also use almond or walnut oil instead.

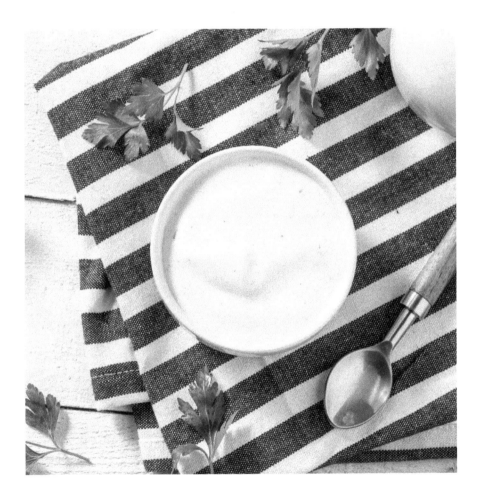

Roasted Lemon Herb Chicken

Ingredients:

12 total pieces bone-in chicken thighs and legs

1 medium onion, thinly sliced

1 tbsp dried rosemary

1 tsp dried thyme

1 lemon, sliced thin

1 orange, sliced thin

For the marinade:

5 tbsp extra virgin olive oil

6 cloves garlic, minced

Stevia to taste

Juice of 1 lemon

Juice of 1 orange

1 tbsp Italian seasoning

1 tsp onion powder

Dash of red pepper flakes

low sodium salt and freshly ground pepper, to taste

Instructions:

Whisk together all of the marinade ingredients in a small bowl. Place the chicken in a baking dish (or a large Ziploc bag) and pour the marinade over it. Marinate for 3 hours to overnight. Preheat the oven to 400 degrees F. Place the chicken in a baking dish and arrange with the onion, orange, and lemon slices. Sprinkle with thyme, rosemary, low sodium salt and pepper. Cover with aluminum foil and bake for 30 minutes. Remove the foil, baste the chicken, and bake for another 30 minutes uncovered, until the chicken is cooked through.

Basil Turkey with Roasted Tomatoes

Ingredients:

1 turkey breasts

1 cup mushrooms, chopped

1/2 medium onion, chopped

1-2 tbsp extra virgin olive oil

Half cup thinly sliced fresh basil

low sodium salt and pepper, to taste

1 pint cherry tomatoes

Stevia to taste

Fresh parsley, for garnish

Instructions:

Preheat the oven to 400 degrees F. Place the tomatoes on a baking sheet and drizzle with olive oil and stevia. Sprinkle with low sodium salt and pepper and toss to coat evenly. Bake for 15-20 minutes until soft. While the tomatoes are roasting, heat one tablespoon of olive oil in a large pan over low heat. Add the onions and mushrooms and cook for 10-12 minutes to soften and caramelize, stirring regularly. Clear a space for the chicken.

Season the turkey with low sodium salt and pepper and then place it in the pan. Simmer for 15 minutes or until the chicken is cooked through. Every 5 minutes or so, spoon the sauce in the pan over the turkey.

To assemble, divide the tomatoes between two plates. Place one turkey breast on each and then spoon the onions, mushrooms, and pan drippings over the turkey. Garnish with parsley.

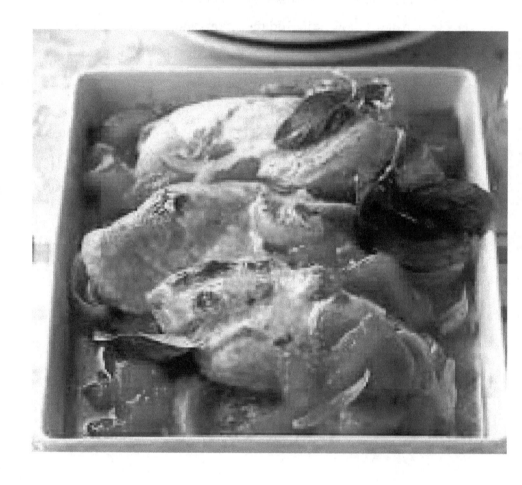

DINNER

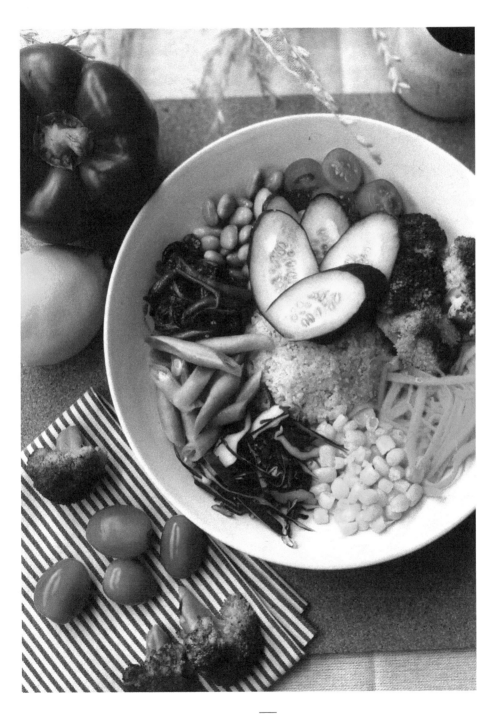

Sexy Shrimp with Delish Veggie Stir Fry

Ingredients:

1 1/2 pounds of shrimp

1 tsp. of coconut oil

1/2 cup of thinly sliced onion

1/2 red bell pepper. thinly sliced

1 cup of full fat coconut milk

2 tbsp. fish sauce

1 tbsp curry powder

2 tbsp. of chopped cilantro

Instructions:

In a large bowl mix fish sauce, garlic and ginger.

Heat the olive oil in a wok (or a large nonstick skillet) over medium-high heat.

Once it starts to shimmer add onion and chiles. Stir-fry the onions until they start to brown around the edges, about 2 minutes.

Stir in the bok choy stems and stir-fry for 1 minute.

Add the beaten eggs and cook until it's nearly cooked through about 2 minutes, stirring often. Stir in bok choy greens, basil and lime juice.

And stir-fry for 30 seconds or so, until the greens are wilted. Serve immediately.

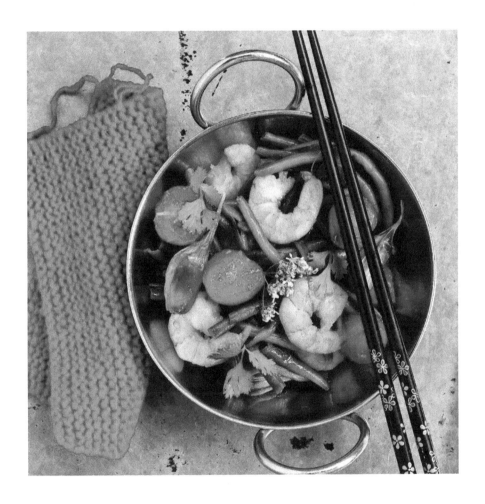

Sexy Spicy Salmon

Ingredients:

Stevia to taste

1 1/2 lemons, juice of

1/2 tsp garlic powder

3 tbsp soy sauce, reduced sodium gluten free

14 oz wild salmon fillets, cut into 4 pieces

1 clove crushed garlic

1 tbsp chilli flakes

7 oz sliced shiitake mushrooms

1 tbsp fresh ginger, finely minced

1 cup snap peas

1/2 cup sliced scallions, divided

1 tbsp black sesame seeds

Instructions:

Mix stevia, juice of half a lemon, garlic powder, and 1 tbsp of the soy sauce in bowl. Add salmon to marinade and set aside in refrigerator up to 30 minutes turning once after 15 minutes; reserve the marinade. Add the remaining

Turkey Stockbroth

Ingredients:

2 tablespoons coconut oil

1 medium onion, diced

2 cloves garlic, minced

1 pound turkey BONES

1 tablespoon coconut amino

10 cups chicken broth

1/4 teaspoon salt

1/4 teaspoon pepper

4 cups fresh spinach leaves, coarsely chopped

Fresh rosemary, optional

Instructions:

Heat the coconut oil in a large stockpot over high heat. Add the onion and garlic and sauté for 2 minutes. Add the ground turkey and sauté for an additional 7 minutes.

Add the coconut amines. Stir frequently for 2 minutes.

Add the chicken broth, salt, and pepper. Simmer for about 20 minutes.

Add the spinach and rosemary (if desired) and sauté for 2 minutes.

Baked Sweet Potato Chips

Ingredients:

2 large sweet potatoes

2 tbsp melted coconut oil

2 tsp dried rosemary

1 tsp sea salt

Instructions:

Preheat oven to 375 degrees F. Peel sweet potatoes and slice thinly, using either a mandolin or sharp knife. In a large bowl, toss sweet potatoes with coconut oil, rosemary, and salt.

Place sweet potato chips in a single layer on a rimmed baking sheet covered with parchment paper. Bake in the oven for 10 minutes, then flip the chips over and bake for another 10 minutes. For the last ten minutes, watch the chips closely and pull off any chips that start to brown, until all of the chips are cooked.

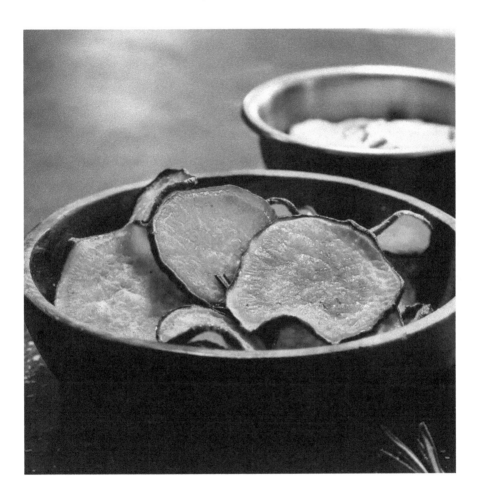

Homemade Paleo Ketchup with a Kick

Ingredients:

1 12 oz can tomato paste

1 cup water

2 tbsp vinegar

½ tsp salt

½ tsp curry powder

½ tsp garlic powder

This recipe makes approximately 32 oz of ketchup, or 64 1tbsp servings.

Directions:

Mix all ingredients in a sauce pan and bring to boil on medium-high heat.

Reduce heat to medium-low and simmer while stirring frequently until flavours have blended. (Add more water for thinner ketchup, add less water for thicker) Transfer to a glass jar and cool before serving.

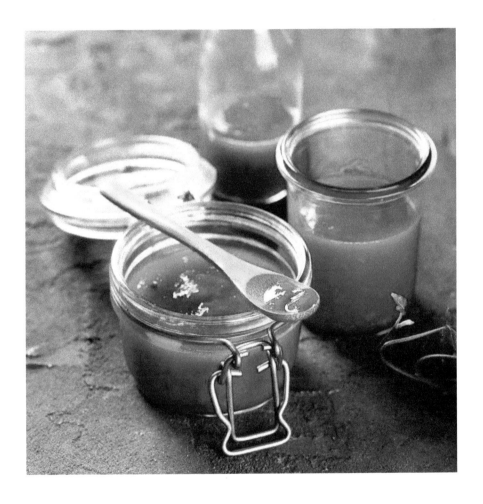

Homemade Paleo Honey Mustard from Scratch

Ingredients:

1/4 cup mustard powder

1/4 cup water

3 tbsp honey

Sea salt, to taste

Instructions:

Place the mustard powder and water in a bowl and stir until combined. Add salt and honey to taste. Let stand for at least 15 minutes before serving.

Red Hot Chicken Broth

Ingredients:

½ red onion, sliced

3 garlic cloves, minced

2 Tbs schmaltz (chicken fat)

1 tsp smoked paprika

½ tsp anchochilli powder or chipotle

1 tsp chilli flakes

1 tsp sea salt

½ tsp fresh cracked pepper

1 large sweet potato, cubed

2 large carrots, cubed

8 C homemade chicken stock

2 kaffir lime leaves (optional)

1 Tbs lime juice

2½ C leftover roast chicken, pulled into bite size chunks green onions for garnish

Instructions:

Heat schmaltz in a large pot, add onion and garlic and cook until onion is translucent. Add spices, salt, sweet potato, carrots and cook for about 2 minutes stirring continuously.

Add chicken stock, lime leaves, lime juice and chicken and allow simmering for 20 minutes.

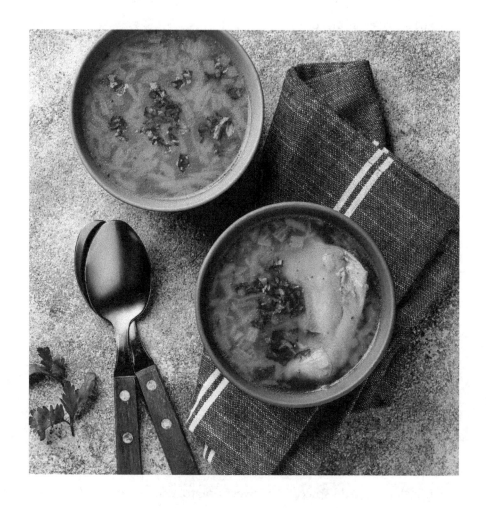

Simple and Easy Chicken Brothstock

Ingredients:

3 kg chicken (Roasted chicken carcasses, chicken wings/winglet's, left over bones from chicken drumsticks)

1 tbsp apple cider vinegar

3 onions

3 carrots

2 sticks of celery

1 tsp peppercorns

5 garlic cloves (unpeeled)

Instructions:

Place the chicken into a very large stock pot and add enough cold water to cover the bones.

Add the cider vinegar and leave the mixture to sit for half an hour.

Roughly chop the onions, carrots and celery.

Place the pan on the heat and add the chopped veg, garlic and peppercorns.

Bring the water to a boil, and then reduce the heat to its very lowest setting and place on a vented lid.

During the first couple of hours use a large spoon to skim off any foam/scum that rises to the top of your stock. This should reduce after the initial cooking period.

Allow the stock to cook at the lowest possible heat for at least 6 hours; 12 hours would be even better.

Remove from the heat and carefully pour the stock through a sieve lined with a clean J-cloth. You will need to do this slowly to ensure you don't dump all the solids back over the side of the sieve and into your stock. Even better would be do to it in 2 or 3 small portions.

Return the stock to the hob, bring to the boil and boil vigorously for 10 minutes.

Your stock is now ready to use in soups, risottos or to freeze for when you need it.

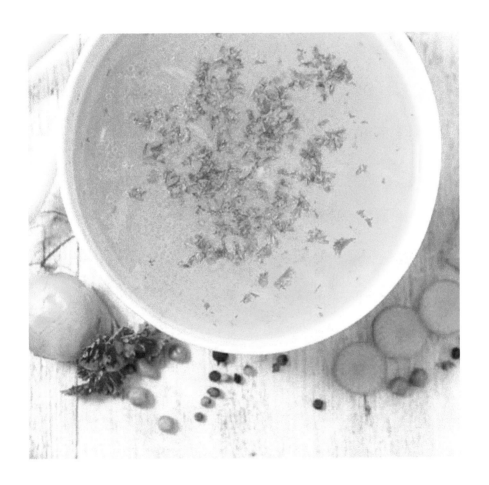

SOUPS

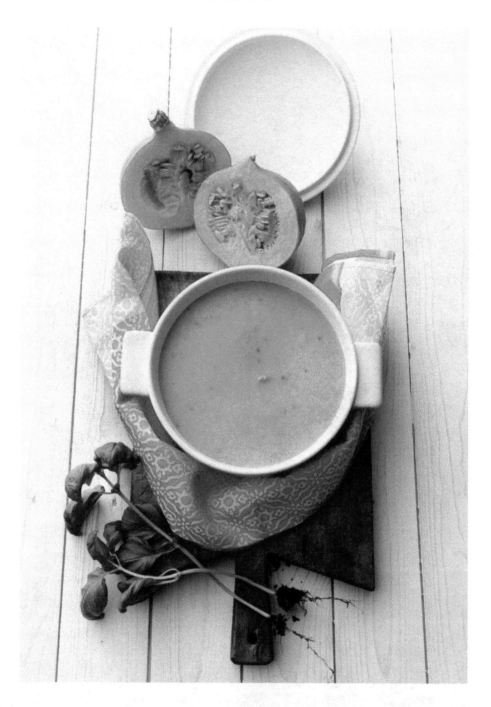

Mighty Andalusian Gazpacho

Ingredients:

3 pounds very ripe tomatoes, cored and cut into chunks

½ pound cucumber, peeled, seeded, and cut chunks

⅓ pound red onion, peeled and cut into chunks

⅓ pound green or red bell pepper, cored, seeded, and cut into chunks

2 cloves garlic, peeled and smashed

1½ teaspoons low sodium salt, plus more to taste

1 cup extra-virgin olive oil, plus more for serving

2 tablespoons sherry vinegar, plus more for serving

2 tablespoons finely minced chives

Freshly ground black pepper

Instructions:

Put all veggies in a large bowl and toss with low sodium salt. Let sit till the veggies have released a lot of their liquid.

Separate the veggies from the liquid, reserving the liquid. Place on a tray and place in the freezer for at least a half hour, or until they are partially frozen.

Remove from freezer and let thaw completely.

Combine the thawed veggies, reserved juice, oil and sherry vinegar in a large bowl. Ladle into a blender, working in batches if necessary, and blend on high until quite smooth. Chill for up to 24 hours.

Serve with extra sherry vinegar, olive oil and a sprinkle of chives

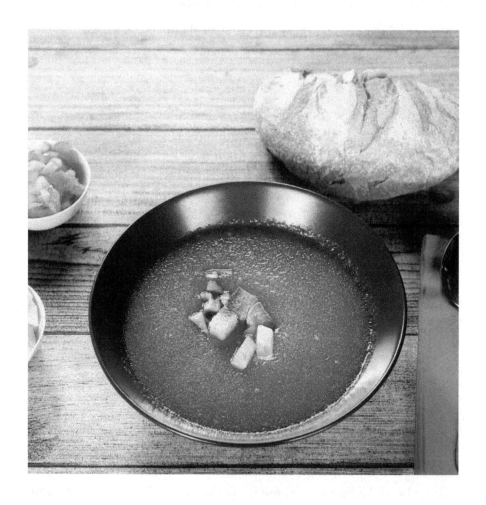

Munchy Mushroom Soup

Ingredients:

500g boneless chicken breast, sliced

150g button, straw or oyster mushrooms

1 large carrots, sliced

4 red tomatoes, quartered

6 cups low sodium chicken stock

2 stalk lemon grass, sliced into 1 cm pieces juice from 4-6 limes (add more if you want it sour) red chillies, chopped

Instructions:

Place the chicken stock in a pot, add lemon grass, and bring to boil over medium heat.

Add the chicken meat, mushrooms, tomatoes, lime juice bring to a boil and simmer for 15 minutes

Add sugar, chillies, carrots and simmer for additional 5 minutes. Serve while hot.

Healthy Chicken Soup

Ingredients:

1 onion

2 carrots

1 celery stick

100g mushrooms

100g frozen peas

1 tbsp butter

1 liter homemade chicken stock

¼ tsp turmeric

1 clove of garlic

Salt and pepper

3 chicken thighs

small handful of parsley

pinch of chilli flakes (optional garnish)

Lemon wedge (optional garnish)

Instructions:

Chop the onion, carrot and celery into fine dice.

Heat the butter in a large pan, add the chopped veg, peas and mushrooms.

Cook gently for 5 minutes.

Add the chicken stock, turmeric and crushed in the garlic.

Taste your stock and add salt and pepper to taste.

Bring to a simmer and add the chicken thighs.

Simmer for 10 minutes until the thighs are cooked through.

Remove the thighs from the liquid and chop into bite sized pieces.

Return the chicken to the soup.

Serve with a sprinkling of fresh parsley.

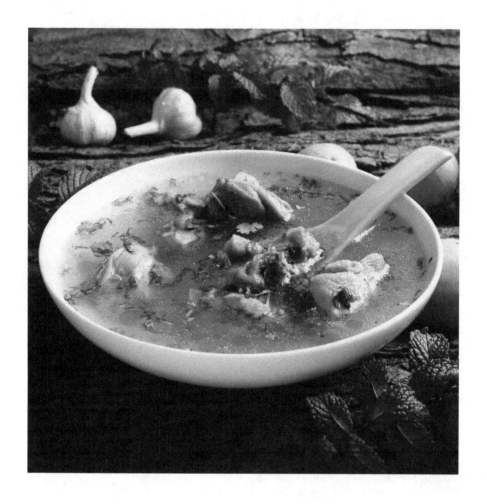

Paleo Crock Pot Chicken Soup

Ingredients:

1 medium onion, chopped

3 celery stalks, diced

3 carrots, diced

1 teaspoon apple cider vinegar

1 tablespoon herbs de Provence, or several sprigs fresh herbs

2 organic chicken breasts, bone-in, skin-on

2 organic chicken thighs, bone-in, skin-on

1 teaspoon sea salt

½ teaspoon fresh ground pepper

3-4 cups filtered water

Instructions:

Layer all ingredients in crock pot in order listed, making sure chicken is bone side down on top of vegetables. Add enough water to cover vegetables and come half way up chicken, between 3 and 4 cups. Cook on low for 6-8 hours.

Remove chicken and let cool slightly. Remove skin and bones. Shred chicken meat and add back to soup in crock pot. Adjust seasonings, reheat, and serve.

Ginger Carrot Delight Soup

Ingredients:

3 tbsp unsalted butter or coconut oil

1 1/2 pounds carrots (6-7 large carrots), sliced

2 cups chopped white or yellow onion

1 cup diced turkey breastlow sodium salt

2 teaspoons minced ginger

2 cups low sodium chicken stock

2 cups water

3 large strips of zest from an orange

Instructions:

Heat up the butter or coconut oil in a large soup pot.

Add the chopped carrots, turkey breast and onion to the pot and cook over medium heat for 5-10 minutes. Don't allow the carrots or onion to brown.

Add in the remaining ingredients (ginger, orange zest, water, and stock). The orange zest will be pulled out prior to puréeing so make sure they are in large, easy to identify strips rather than small pieces. Bring to a boil then simmer for 10 minutes.

Remove orange zest strips. Purée the mixture with an immersion blender. Or divide into 3-4 batches and blend in a regular blender.

I garnished my soup with a touch of olive oil and some freshly ground low sodium salt and pepper.

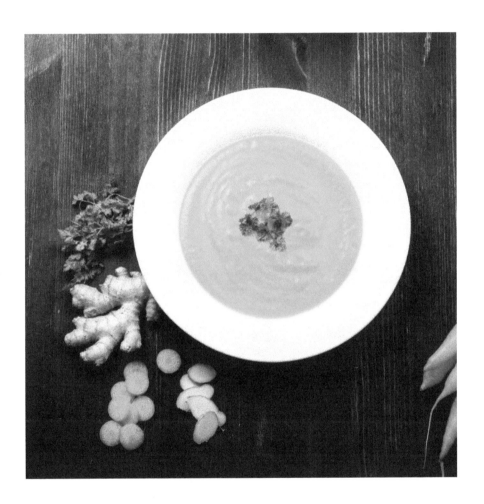

Paleo Chicken Soup

Ingredients:

2 pounds uncooked chicken breasts/thighs

1 pound diced carrots

2 medium sweet potatoes cubed (I love white sweet potatoes!) or 1 pound parsnips diced

6 ribs/stalks celery chopped

1 onion diced

2-3 garlic cloves diced finely

2 to 3 tsp sea salt

1/2 to 1 tsp black pepper

4 cups chopped kale or collards.

6 to 8 cups Chicken Broth/Stock

Optional: 1 to 2 tbsp dried herbs (rosemary, thyme, sage)

Instructions:

Grab your slow cooker or giant stock pot. Add all of ingredients except for the broth.

If you like a thicker soup, add just enough broth to barely cover the ingredients. If you enjoy a more broth-y soup add the full amount of broth. Slow Cooker: 7 to 8 hours on low, 3-4 hours on high. Stovetop: Bring the soup to a boil, cover, and reduce to simmer (low) – leave for one hour.

Once the soup is finished cooking (chicken is cooked through and veggies are soft) remove the chicken and shred or chop it.

Roasted Cauliflower and Sweet Potato Soup

Ingredients:

1 head of cauliflower, chopped into florets

2 medium-sized sweet potatoes, peeled and cubed;

5 garlic cloves, peeled;

1 tsp. paprika; (omit for AIP)

4 cups vegetable or chicken stock;

1/2 cup coconut or almond milk; (coconut for AIP)

2 tbsp. olive oil;

Sea salt and freshly ground black pepper;

Instructions:

Preheat your oven to 400 F.

Place the cauliflower florets, cubed potatoes, and garlic on a baking sheet.

Drizzle with olive oil, and season to taste with salt and pepper.

Roast in the oven for 35 to 40 minutes or until the vegetables are soft.

Transfer the vegetables from the baking sheet to a saucepan.

Pour the vegetable stock into the saucepan, and add the paprika.

Bring to a simmer and purée the soup using an immersion blender.

Pour in the coconut or almond milk, and give everything a good stir.

Continue simmering until warm, and season to taste before serving.

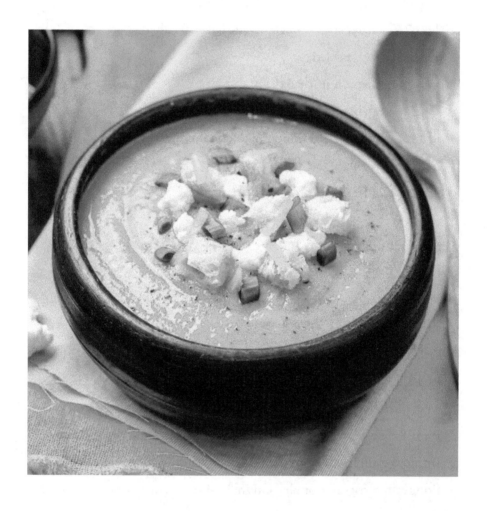

Turkey and Vegetable Soup Recipe

Ingredients:

2 cups leftover turkey, chopped;

1 onion, diced;

3 to 4 carrots, diced;

2 parsnips, diced;

2 celery stalks, diced;

1 cup cauliflower, riced;

1 ½ cups cabbage, shredded;

2 bay leaves;

2 garlic cloves, minced;

2 tsp. ground sage;

1 tsp. thyme;

Sea salt and freshly ground black pepper;

Turkey stock

Ingredients: for Turkey Stock

1 turkey carcass or 5 lbs. turkey parts (preferably bony parts, like necks and backs);

2 yellow onions, quartered;

2 celery ribs, cut into big chunks;

2 carrots, cut into big chunks;

4 garlic cloves;

4 sprigs fresh thyme;

1 bay leave;

4 quarts cold water;

Freshly ground black pepper;

Instructions:

Place the turkey carcass or parts in a saucepan, add all the remaining ingredients for the stock, and season to taste with pepper.

Fill the saucepan with water and bring to a boil.

Lower heat to a light simmer, and simmer 4 to 8 hours. (adding water if necessary).

Strain the stock with a fine mesh sieve, throwing away all the remaining ingredients. Set aside the stock for now.

Pick through the carcass. Remove any meat you find, and add it to the meat for the soup. Add all the ingredients for the soup in a large saucepan. Fill the pan with the turkey stock, and season to taste.

Bring to a simmer, and simmer 45 minutes to 1 hour.

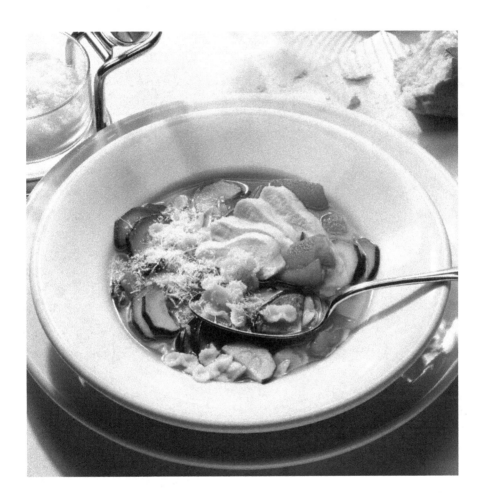

DESSERTS

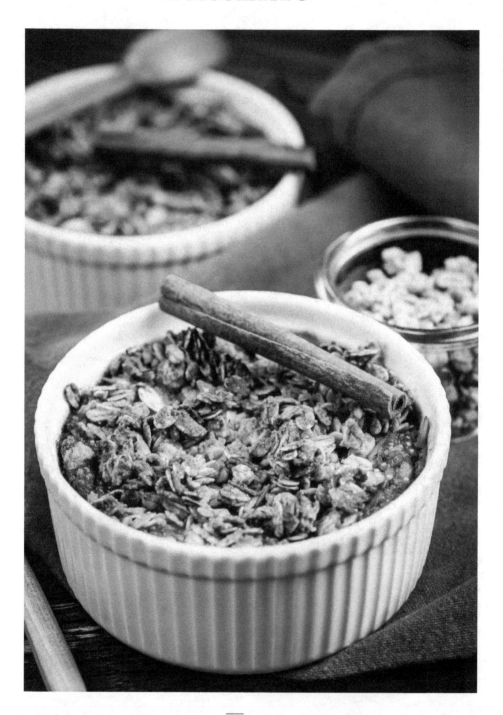

Choco – Almond Delights

Ingredients:

1 c. toasted hazelnuts

1 c. raw almonds

2/3 c. raw almond butter

5 Tbs. raw cacao powder (or unsweetened cocoa powder)

1/2 tsp. vanilla extract

1/4 c. unsweetened, shredded coconut

Instructions:

Combine all the ingredients, except for the coconut, in the food processor. Whir until smooth. This will take a few minutes and may require scraping down the sides of the bowl one or more times. Line a mini muffin tin with plastic wrap. Spoon dollops of the sweet mixture into the lined tin cups and form into "mounds." Freeze until well formed. Remove mounds from plastic and tin and flip for presentation. Sprinkle with shredded coconut.

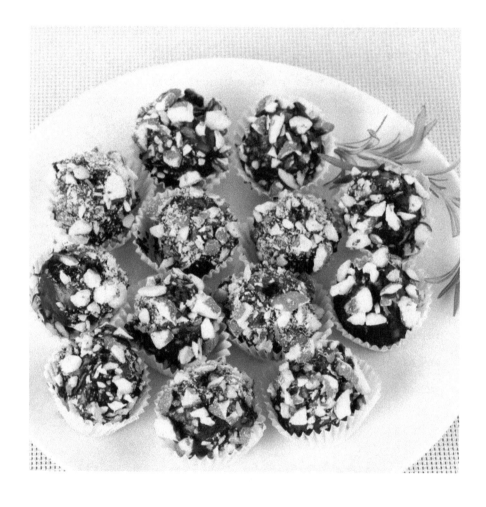

Fetching Fudge

Ingredients:

1 cup coconut butter

1/4 cup coconut oil

1/4 cup cocoa

1/4 cup cocoa powder + 1 Tbsp

Stevia to taste

1 tsp vanilla

Instructions:

In the pot, gently melt the cocoa butter on low (number 2)

When it is half melted add the butter, the coconut oil and the coconut spread and gently mix with the whisk as it melts

Add vanilla, and stevia and whisk in well

Add the cocoa powder and whisk in well

Be sure to take the pot off the heat when the fat is melted and keep whisking until it is smooth and all the lumps are out — you don't want to overheat this

Pour into the 8 x 8 pan that is lined with parchment paper

Refrigerate for 1 – 2 hours

When solid, pull the parchment paper out of the pan, put the block of fudge on a flat surface and cut into small squares

Enjoy! This will melt rather quickly — but it won't last long!

Coco – Walnut Brownie Bites

Ingredients:

2/3 cup raw walnut halves and pieces

1/3 cup unsweetened cocoa powder

1 tablespoon vanilla extract

1 to 2 tablespoons coconut milk

2/3 cups shredded unsweetened coconut

Instructions:

Pulse coconut in food processor for 30 seconds to a minute to form coconut crumbs. Remove from food processor and set aside. Add unsweetened cocoa powder and walnuts to food processor, blend until walnuts become fine crumbs, but do not over process or you will get some kind of chocolate walnut butter. Place in the food processor the cocoa walnut crumbs. Add vanilla. Process until mixture starts to combine. Add coconut milk. You will know the consistency is right when the dough combines into a ball in the middle of the food processor. If dough is too runny add a tablespoon or more cocoa powder to bring it back to a dough like state. Transfer dough to a bowl and cover with plastic wrap. Refrigerate for at least 2 hours. Cold dough is much easier to work with. I left my dough in the fridge over night. You could put it in the freezer if you need to speed the process up. Roll the dough balls in coconut crumbs, pressing the crumbs gently into the ball. Continue until all dough is gone.

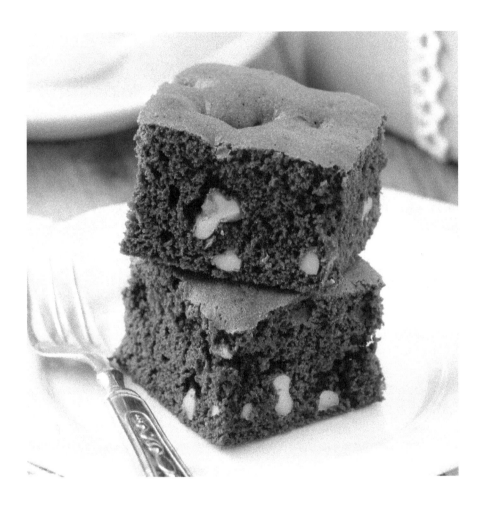

Choco-coco Brownies

Ingredients:

6 Tablespoons of coconut oil

6 ounces of Sugar free Chocolate

4 Tablespoons of Packed Coconut Flour (20g)

¼ cup of Unsweetened Cocoa Powder (30g)

2 Eggs

½ teaspoon of Baking Soda

¼ teaspoon of low sodium salt

Extra coconut oil for pan greasing

Stevia to taste

Instructions:

Preheat the oven to 350F. Grease an 8x8 baking pan and line with parchment paper.

Ensure eggs are at room temperature. You may run them under warm water for about 10 seconds while shelled.

Gently melt the semisweet chocolate and oil in a double boiler. You may use the microwave at 50% heat at 30 second intervals with intermittent stirring.

Stir in unsweetened cocoa powder.

Sift together the superfine coconut flour, baking soda, stevia and low sodium salt. Beat the eggs and add the dry ingredients. Beat until combined Add the rest of the wet ingredients and beat until incorporated.

Pour the batter into the lined 8x8 pan.

Bake for 25-30 minutes at 350F until a toothpick inserted into the center of the batter comes out clean.

When done, remove from the oven and let cool in the pan for at least 15 minutes.

Delicious Coconut Flour Cake with Strawberry Surprise

Ingredients:

1 dozen eggs

2 cups coconut milk (I used homemade)

¼ cup milk

2 teaspoons Stevia

2 teaspoons vanilla extract

2 cups coconut flour

1/2 teaspoon baking soda

1/4 teaspoon low sodium salt coconut oil for greasing the pan

Instructions:

Preheat oven to 350F.

Whisk together the eggs, coconut milk, milk, stevia and vanilla extract. Mix until smooth.

Add coconut flour, baking soda and salt to the egg mixture and whisk until a smooth batterforms.

Grease 2 – 9 inch round cake pans with coconut oil.

Divide up the batter evenly between the 2 cake tins. Use a rubber spatula to smooth it out.

Bake for 40 minutes, or until a toothpick inserted into the center of the cake comes out clean.

Allow the cake to cool.

Fill the center with cooked strawberries (recipe below). You can also use the strawberry fillingto decorate the cake.

Strawberry Filling

Ingredients:

2 cups organic strawberries, stems removed and sliced

Place the strawberries in a saucepan over medium heat.

After a few minutes, the strawberries will release their juices.

Allow them to cook uncovered, occasionally stirring and smashing them. Keep cooking them until the strawberries are soft, smashed and the sauce has reduced.About 30 minutes.

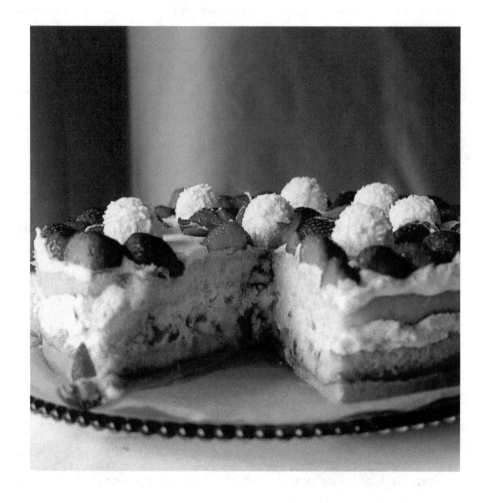

Titillating Berry Trifle

Ingredients:

1/2 cup plus 2 tsp coconut flour, sifted

1/4 tsp low sodium salt

1/4 tsp baking soda

5 whole eggs (2 of them separated)

1/2 cup coconut oil, softened

1/2 cup almond milk

2 tsp stevia

1 tablespoon vanilla extract

2 teaspoons lemon juice

1 1/2-2 cups washed & diced strawberries (cut large if using a traditional Trifle bowl)

1 1/2-2 cups washed blueberries

1 1/2-2 cups washed raspberries

3-4 cans full-fat coconut milk, cream only

Instructions:

Preheat oven to 350 degrees.

Sift the dry ingredients together and set aside.

Separate 2 of the eggs, setting the whites aside and putting the 2 yolks in a medium sizedbowl. Crack open the rest of the eggs, adding them to the bowl with egg yolks.

Sexy Savory Muffins

Ingredients:

½ cup coconut flour

1 tsp baking soda

½-1 tsp low sodium salt

¼ cup coconut oil

½ cup + 2 tbsp coconut milk

4 pastured eggs

1 tsp apple cider vinegar

1 tsp garlic powder

½ tsp each of rosemary, thyme, sage

Instructions:

Pre-heat the oven to 350°. Melt the coconut oil and combine with remaining muffin ingredients in a food processor or bowl, mix well.

Place batter in a muffin tin lined with muffin liners. The muffins will raise a small amount, soyou can fill the muffin liner about ¾ full–almost to the top. Bake for about 20-30 minutes or until a toothpick inserted comes out clean and the tops are slightly browned.

Let it cool and slice in small squares.

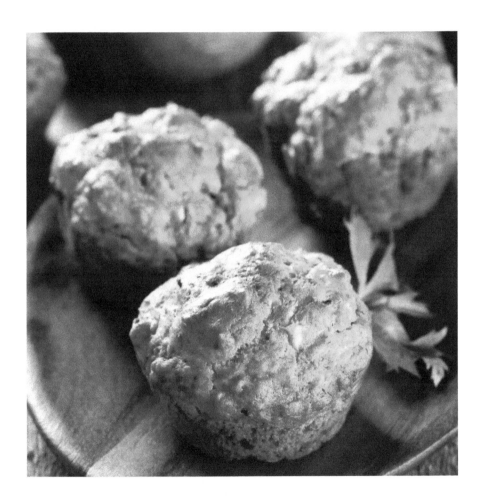

Delicious Lady Fingers

Ingredients:

4 Pastured Eggs, separated

1/4 cup almond milk

1/4 tsp Baking Soda

1/2 tsp Pure Vanilla Extract

1/3 cup Coconut Flour, sifted

1 tsp freshly ground Coffee

Instructions:

Preheat oven to back at 400 degrees.

Beat egg whites until stiff in a standing kitchen mixer, or with a hand mixer.

In a medium sized mixing bowl, combine egg yolks, baking soda, vanilla extract, and milk.

Whisk until combined.

Sift in the coconut flour, and continue to whisk until smooth.

Fold in the egg whites, followed by the coffee grounds.

On a parchment lined baking sheet pipe out 3 inch long cookies with a round piping tube.

Bake at 400 degrees for 13 minutes, or until cookies are golden brown.

Allow to cool and enjoy.

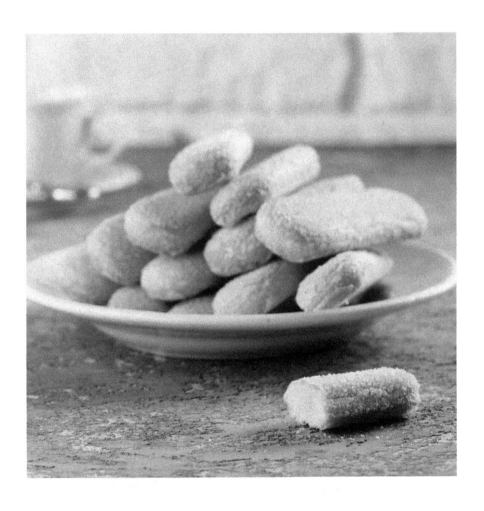

BEVERAGES AND SNACKS

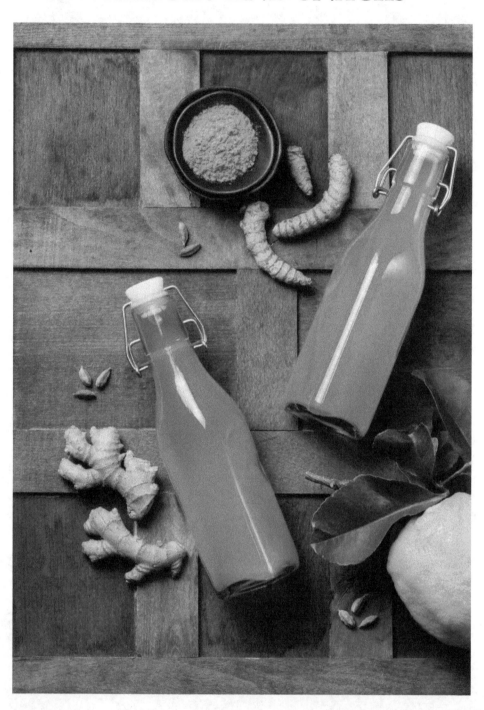

Easy Paleo Shepherd's Pie

For the top layer

1 large head cauliflower, cut into florets

2 tbsp ghee, melted

1 tsp spicy Paleo mustard

Salt and freshly ground black pepper, to taste

Fresh parsley, to garnish

For the bottom layer

1 tbsp coconut oil

1/2 large onion, diced

3 carrots, diced

2 celery stalks, diced

1 lb. lean ground beef

2 tbsp tomato paste

1 cup chicken broth

1 tsp dry mustard

1/4 tsp cinnamon

1/8 tsp ground clove

Salt and freshly ground black pepper, to taste

Instructions:

Place a couple inches of water in a large pot. Once the water is boiling, place steamer insert and then cauliflower florets into the pot and cover. Steam for 12-14 minutes, until tender. Drain and return cauliflower to the pot.

Add the ghee, mustard, salt, and pepper to the cauliflower. Using an immersion blender or food processor, combine the ingredients until smooth. Set aside.

Meanwhile, heat the coconut oil in a large skillet over medium heat. Add the onion, celery, and carrots and sauté for 5 minutes. Add in the ground beef and cook until browned.

Stir the tomato paste, chicken broth, and remaining spices into the meat mixture. Season to taste with salt and pepper. Simmer until most of the liquid has evaporated, about 8 minutes, stirring occasionally. Distribute the meat mixture evenly among four ramekins and spread the pureed cauliflower on top. Use a fork to create texture in the cauliflower and drizzle with olive oil. Place under the broiler for 5-7 minutes until the top turns golden. Sprinkle with fresh parsley and serve.

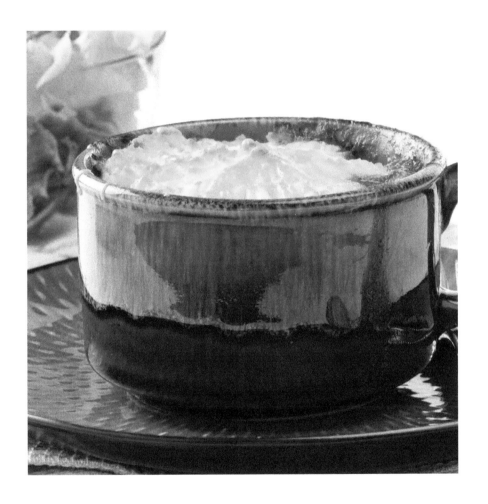

Spicy Avocado Dill Dressing

Ingredients:

1 very ripe avocado

2 tablespoons olive oil

3 sprigs fresh dill

1 tbsp chili powder (more or less to taste)

1 tbsp lime juice

1 tbsp honey

2 tbsp apple cider vinegar

2 cloves garlic

¼ cup almond milk

¼ cup water

Directions:

Combine all ingredients in a blender, process until creamy.

Store in an airtight jar or container in refrigerator, will last

Ginger Carrot Protein Smoothie

Ingredients:

3/4 cup carrot juice

1 tablespoon hemp protein powder

1 tablespoon hulled hemp seeds

1/2 apple

3 to 4 ice cubes

1/2 inch piece fresh ginger

Instructions:

Add to a blender and blend until smooth.

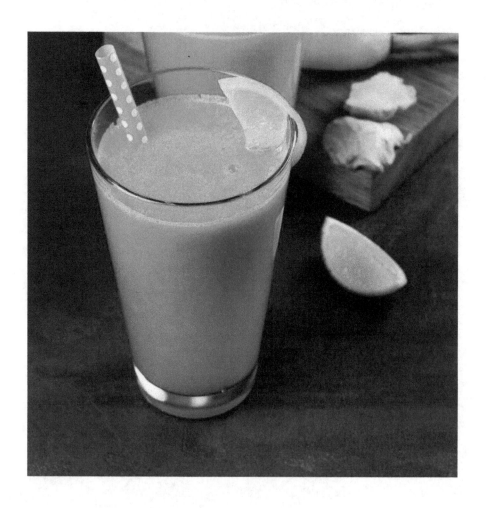

Tropical Green Smoothie

Ingredients:

1 C raw kale, washed and chopped

1 banana, frozen

½ C mango chunks, frozen

½ C pineapple chunks, frozen

1 C coconut water

Instructions:

Add all ingredients to blender and blend on high speed until smooth (takes about 30 seconds.)

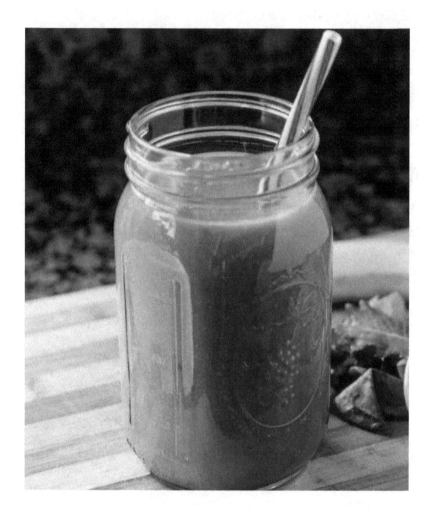

Low Carb Fried Zucchini

Ingredients::

3 medium zucchini or yellow squash

2 eggs

1 tablespoon water

1/3 cup coconut flour

1/4 cup powdered

Parmesan cheese

vegetable oil, for frying

ranch dressing, for serving

Directions::

Heat a 1/4 inch of oil in the bottom of a large skillet over medium heat. Wash and slice the zucchini into thin rounds, about 1/8-1/4 inch thick. Beat together the egg and water in a shallow bowl.

Stir together the coconut flour and Parmesan in a second shallow bowl. Coat the zucchini in the egg and then dredge in the coconut mixture to coat. Add a single layer of zucchini to the hot oil, being careful not to crowd the pan. Fry for 1-2 minutes on each side, until golden brown. Repeat with remaining zucchini.

Drain on a paper towel lined plate. Sprinkle with salt, if desired. Serve with ranch dressing for dipping.

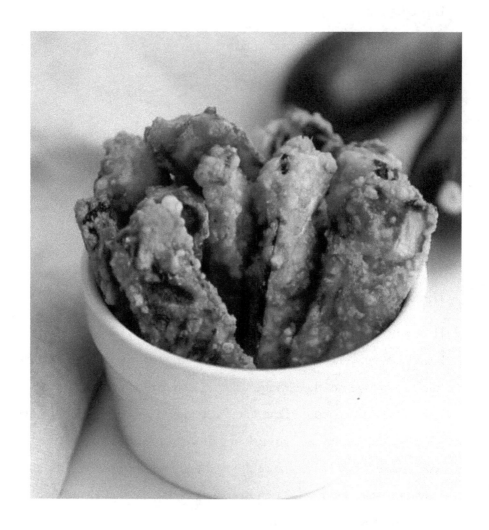

Easy Garlic Butter Spread

Ingredients:

1/2 cup softened Butter

1 tsp Garlic Powder

1/4 tsp Onion Powder

1/2 tsp Dried Parsley

Directions:

Mix together ingredients until well blended Spread on top of sliced bread (I used French) Broil on low until browned.

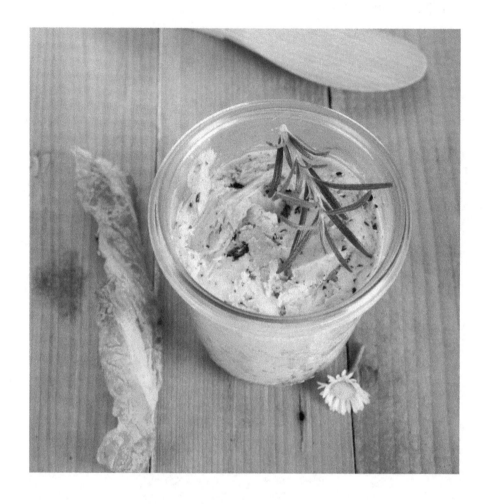

High Protein and Nutritional Delish Smoothie

Ingredients:

1 cup almond milk

1/2 Avocado

4 Strawberries

1/2 Bananas (Very ripe)

1/2 cup Raw Kale or spinach

1/4 cup Carrot or 100 % Orange Juice (legal) (water can be subbed)

1 cup Coconut Yogurt..or almond milk)

1 tablespoon hemp protein powder

Instructions:

Add everything to your blender, More water or ice can be added to help with your preferred texture/thickness.

Pineapple Protein Smoothie

Ingredients:

1 cup (135g) pineapple chunks

1 cup (200g) coconut milk (fresh or tinned)

½ med (65g) banana

¼ cup (65g) ice cubes

¼ tsp vanilla bean powder

pinch low sodium salt

1 tablespoon hemp protein powder

Instructions:

Peel pineapple and chop into small chunks.

Put everything into a high speed blender and blend until smooth.

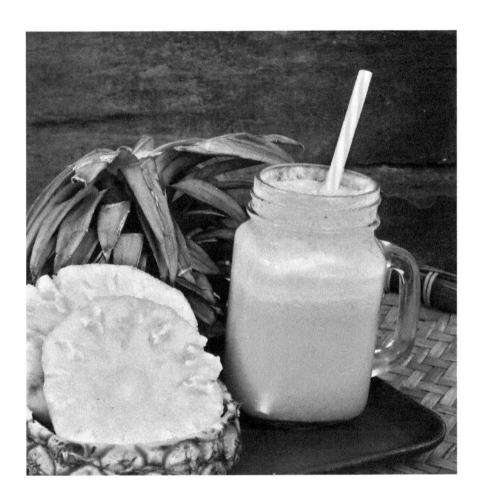

SUSAN MULLER